THE COMBATIVE PERSPECTIVE

THE COMBATIVE PERSPECTIVE

The Thinking Man's Guide to Self-Defense

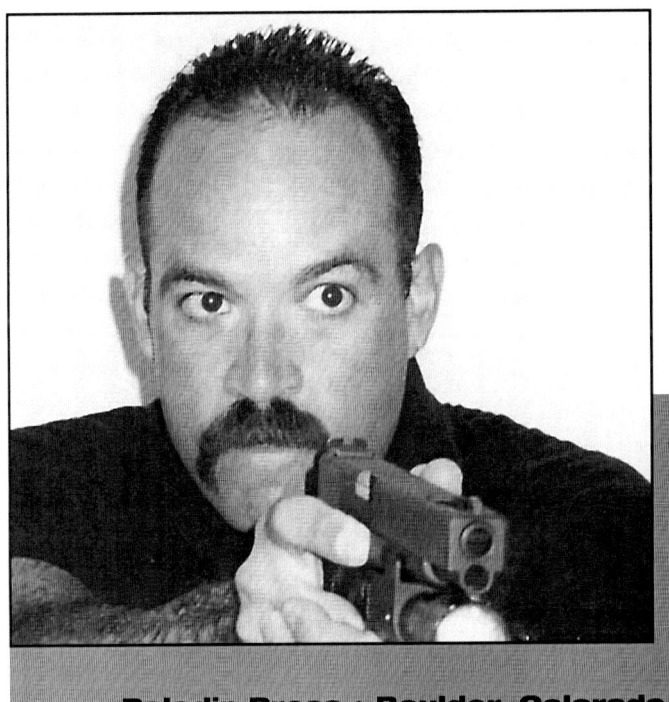

Paladin Press • Boulder, Colorado

Also by Gabriel Suarez:

Close-Range Gunfighting (video)
Force-on-Force Gunfight Training
The Tactical Advantage
The Tactical Advantage: The Video
The Tactical Pistol (also available in Spanish)
Tactical Pistol Marksmanship
Tactical Rifle

The Combative Perspective:
The Thinking Man's Guide to Self-Defense
by Gabe Suarez

Copyright © 2003 by Gabe Suarez

ISBN 10: 1-58160-404-1
ISBN 13: 978-1-58160-404-7
Printed in the United States of America

Published by Paladin Press, a division of
Paladin Enterprises, Inc.
Gunbarrel Tech Center
7077 Winchester Circle
Boulder, Colorado 80301 USA
+1.303.443.7250

Direct inquiries and/or orders to the above address.

PALADIN, PALADIN PRESS, and the "horse head" design are trademarks belonging to Paladin Enterprises and registered in United States Patent and Trademark Office.

All rights reserved. Except for use in a review, no portion of this book may be reproduced in any form without the express written permission of the publisher.

Neither the author nor the publisher assumes any responsibility for the use or misuse of information contained in this book.

Visit our Web site at www.paladin-press.com

To my brother in arms, Dale Fricke.
I cannot thank him enough for bringing me fresh
ammunition and for pointing out the
right direction during "the fog of war."

And for my other brothers in arms,
members of the elite 15 percent who
counted with me in the dark places of the earth.

Blessed be the Lord my Rock
who trains my hands for war,
and my fingers for battle.
—Psalm 144:1

If you can keep your head when all about you
Are losing theirs and blaming it on you;
If you can trust yourself when all men doubt you,
But make allowance for their doubting too;
If you can wait and not be tired of waiting,
Or, being lied about, don't deal in lies,
Or, being hated, don't give way to hating,
And yet don't look too good, nor talk too wise;

If you can dream—and not make dreams your master;
If you can think—and not make thoughts your aim;
If you can meet with triumph and disaster
And treat those two impostors just the same;
If you can bear to hear the truth you've spoken
Twisted by knaves to make a trap for fools,
Or watch the things you gave your life to, broken,
And stoop to build 'em up with worn out tools;

If you can make one heap of all your winnings
And risk it on one turn of pitch-and-toss,
And lose, and start again at your beginnings
And never breathe a word about your loss;
If you can force your heart and nerve and sinew
To serve you long after they are gone,
And so hold on when there is nothing in you
Except the Will which says to them: "Hold On";

If you can talk with crowds and keep your virtue,
Or walk with kings—nor lose the common touch;
If neither foes nor loving friends can hurt you;
If all men count with you, but none too much;
If you can fill the unforgiving minute
With sixty seconds worth of distance run—
Yours is the Earth and everything that's in it,
And—which is more—you'll be a man, my son!

—Rudyard Kipling

Table of Contents

PREFACE xi

INTRODUCTION 1

DESIRE FOR VICTORY | PART ONE **11**

   1. WHAT DESIRE IS MADE OF 13

ELIMINATION OF UNCERTAINTY | PART TWO **19**

   2. LIABILITY 23

   3. THE NATURE AND INTENT OF THE ADVERSARY 41

   4. VICTIM OR VICTOR? ATTITUDE IS EVERYTHING 45

SITUATIONAL AWARENESS | PART THREE **65**

   5. COOPER'S MENTAL TRIGGER 69

   6. THE OODA LOOP 75

WILLINGNESS TO ACT | PART FOUR **85**

   7. ON COURAGE: REFUTING THE "NEW CONSCIOUSNESS" 89

A FINAL WORD 95

ABOUT THE AUTHOR 97

Preface

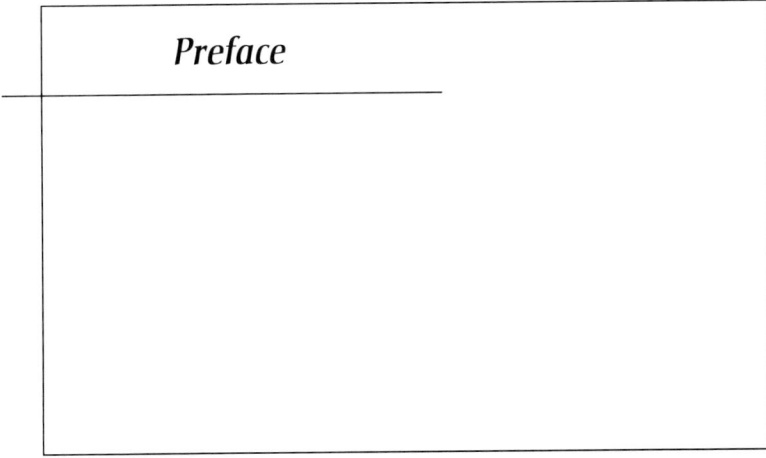

First of all, I want to thank you for your continued support. I often say to my clients that without students there would be no teachers. Much the same can be said about the relationship between writers and readers.

Those of you who've read my other works will notice that there is something quite different about this book. Even the title is different. Most of my other works have focused on the actual operational issues of weapons and their specific tactical deployment. In *The Combative Perspective*, I'm not writing about the latest CQB technique or the best way to deploy a shotgun or even a newly discovered way to sneak around in the darkness looking for hostiles.

This book is not about developing better skills with your weapons. Quite to the contrary, this entire volume is devoted solely to developing your knowledge about and properly organizing your mental attitude toward

The Combative Perspective

combative encounters. It is intended to develop your thinking and your spirit in the realm of what can jokingly be referred to, in Pentagon-ese, as "Close Range Inter-Personal Confrontations." In other words, fights. The contents are as applicable to the bladesman as they are to the rifleman, and to the unarmed fighter as they are to the pistolero.

In *The Tactical Advantage*, I wrote that even the world's best gunfighter will get killed if he exercises poor tactics. Likewise, a dramatic and glorious demise is the prize for the man who does not know what he's doing, does not have a plan already thought out, or simply has the wrong mental attitude.

In my years "downrange" working as a police officer and protection specialist, I found that the right mental attitude, even if the odds were clearly against you, often won the day. On the contrary, even the best-equipped and (supposedly) trained SWAT teams lost if their minds were not "right."

"Getting your mind right," as one of my original training officers used to say, involves a certain attitude about life and death and a certain outlook on the world. These things, however, are not easily taught in school. They are things that the individual must cultivate and develop mentally and spiritually. This book will lead you through the thought process that helps to develop this kind of attitude and outlook.

I've included many lessons learned from statistics. Obtained from diverse sources, these statistics help paint a picture of what (and whom) you are likely to

Preface

face. I've also included an interview that I conducted a number of years ago with a real-life bad guy, hours after an incident where he was shot in a home-invasion robbery. Finally, I've incorporated discussions on home defense and mental concepts such as the color code of readiness, Col. Jeff Cooper's "mental trigger," and Col. John Boyd's OODA Loop. Above all, the book is interlaced with my observations from more than 15 years of actual operational experience.

My sole concern is to show you what it takes to win (not just to survive) a fight. I've never made concessions for so-called political correctness (I prefer to call that loathsome but increasingly popular concept "institutional cowardice"), and I certainly will not do so now.

Fights—real fights—are ugly, bloody events that can only be won with ugly and bloody methods. There will never be a referee to call foul or an attorney to advise the culprit of his maleficence. Nor is anyone likely to come to your aid. To the contrary, people will stand by and watch you bleed to death in the gutter as if it were some sort of *Real TV* episode.

If you have sensitive nerves or are excessively tender of heart, put the book away and go watch some nice, sedate daytime talk show. I have pulled no punches here, and I have called the proverbial spade by its proper name. I offer no apologies for that. Undoubtedly, the contents will offend some and shock others. The truth sometimes does that.

Much the same can be said about my discussion of the pervasive, unreasonable fear of the legal repercus-

The Combative Perspective

sions of winning a fight. Some noted writers and police administrators have made lucrative careers of frightening the willies out of those who would hold off the savages by force. ("Let's allow them to kill us so we will not risk being sued!") I find it remarkable that these same fellows have yet to actually hear—much less see—a shot fired in anger. They have never had to fight for their lives, nor have they ever faced the repercussions of the out-of-control legal system they write so prolifically about.

Although this book will address some of these legal and civil issues, its focus is the most important mission, which is to WIN THE FIGHT. After you've won, everything else will find its proper balance.

Much of this information has never been offered in this context before, and I believe that it will be invaluable to the reader as it has been to me during my years in service (perhaps to the unending regret of my adversaries . . . on both sides of the fence).

So grab a comfortable chair, pour yourself a cool adult beverage, light up a nice Partagas, and start turning the pages. I promise that the trip will be astounding and educational, but above all, it will be entertaining.

Strength and Honor,

Gabe Suarez
Prescott, Arizona

Introduction

There is a great deal more to developing the capability to <u>win a violent fight</u> than simply becoming a good fighter or gaining an understanding of tactics. Notice, first of all, that I said *win*, and not *survive*. It has been popular in the writings of many of my colleagues to claim that there are no winners in a fight, only survivors. This is pure nonsense. You can be riddled with bullets or slashed into an unrecognizable shred of blood and tissue and survive, but who wants that? We want to win, pure and simple. This desire is the first requirement of what I call *the combative perspective*. If you don't have it or cannot accept that, then put your hands back in your pockets and hope that you "survive." The rest of us want to win.

Part of the combative perspective is what has been called "mind-set." Mind-set is a good term, but it doesn't cover all of the issues that we need to address. There are

The Combative Perspective

four basic components to the combative perspective: desire for victory, elimination of uncertainty, development of situational awareness, and willingness to act. We've already touched on the desire for victory. Let's look at the other components.

The Chinese tactician Sun Tsu wrote in his classic book *The Art of War* that if we know ourselves and know the enemy, there is no danger in any battle. Any battle is, of course, dangerous, but what Sun Tsu meant by danger was "uncertainty." If there is any uncertainty in your mind, there will be a great deal of hesitation, because you don't know where you stand. Hesitation on your part gives the adversary a definite advantage because while you are debating, he is acting. With hesitation, then, there is a great deal of danger. This is as true today as it was in the days of swords and spears. By eliminating uncertainty you will minimize hesitation and, in doing so, minimize the danger that comes from it.

What are some of the issues that a modern warrior might be uncertain about?

For many, one of the gravest concerns revolves around questions of liability. In eliminating this uncertainty, it is essential to have a full understanding of the rules of engagement. By rules of engagement I mean, of course, the directives, policies, or laws under which you operate. Everyone has these lines beyond which they cannot go. The soldier and the police officer have rules about whom they can engage, as does the civilian. It is particularly important for the former two to have a

Introduction

firm understanding of these rules because most modern institutions (police or military) will not hesitate to sacrifice one of their own if it is considered expedient to do so.

Although some of these rules are very clear, others can be ambiguous. When I first began my professional career, we had the following list of events for determining when we could shoot:

An officer may use deadly force to

1) defend himself from a threat of deadly force or great bodily injury,
2) defend another officer from the same,
3) defend a citizen from the same,
4) prevent a crime involving the use or threatened use of deadly force, or
5) apprehend a suspect of a crime involving the use or threatened use of deadly force.

This was all very clear, and as soon as we received a radio call, we knew whether it fell within one of these categories. When we arrived on scene, there was little hesitation because there was no uncertainty. Today the simple rules take up more than five pages of nebulous written text that requires a separate instructional booklet to be issued to the troops so they can "understand" what the policy means. In short, the "powers that run things" have made things so confusing for the officers that the uncertainty of action is very high.

The Combative Perspective

For the soldier, it may be much clearer: if the other fellow is wearing a different uniform, he's usually good to go.

The private citizen/civilian may, if necessary, act as a policeman would act. More often, however, a civilian acts only in his own defense or in defense of his immediate group or family. It is imperative that he has a clear understanding of the statutes in his region covering the justifiable use of deadly force.

In general, throughout the civilized world, self-defense is accepted as a reason to deploy deadly force (from fists to firearms). If you live in an area that does not believe in personal self-defense, I can't help you. You can either be a live criminal, a defiant freeman, or a dead but legal citizen. Or, of course, you can move away.

In our lectures and courses, we use the acronym IDOL (Immediate Defense of Life) to describe a formula that covers just about every instance where deadly force is justifiable for self-defense. It's easy to remember and even easier to apply. Few places in the world would argue against the pure logic and moral reasoning behind this concept. In applying this formula, the civilian (and perhaps the police officer as well) asks himself, "If I do not act, will someone die or be seriously injured?" If the answer is yes, then he must take care of business! (We will discuss IDOL in greater depth in Part Two.)

Once that last shot has been fired, there is a possibility of facing judicial, administrative, civil, or journalistic persecution for having won. Unfortunately, sometimes the world is run by cowards who could never do

Introduction

what you did, and the very fact that people like you exist makes them nervous. To eliminate the uncertainty of combat blowback, you must understand your legal rules of engagement, protect your financial assests, and have a support structure in place in the event that the cowards with pencils come looking for you. Preparation may not eliminate uncertainty, but it will make eventualities easier to handle.

If you understand your rules of engagement and how to avoid (or at least deal with) the entanglements that might follow, there will be little or no uncertainty in that aspect of things and, therefore, minimal danger.

Another part of the picture that holds a great deal of uncertainty is the nature and intentions of the adversary (in our case, the criminal/terrorist). In wartime, or in a special police application, there is often ample time to develop intelligence on the opponent. It would be nice to learn his strengths and weaknesses, as well as the nature of his intentions . . . and while we are at it, why not also get a Xerox copy of his plans of action?

In the dynamic confrontations of the police officer or civilian defender, there is little time to do much more than determine that there is a fight in progress. The adversary often dictates the time, and even the battlefield, for the confrontation.

Still, although there are always exceptions, we can learn a great deal about our criminal adversaries by studying other criminals. During my formative years, I had the dubious opportunity to work as a deputy sheriff in jail facilities of various levels. I learned a great

The Combative Perspective

deal about my future opponents as well as their methods and motivations.

I'm not suggesting that you hang out in jails, but there are many resources available that document the counterculture's methods and motivations. With the resources available on the Internet, all you need to do is look for them. Learn from and study your enemy, because he is doing the same.

As a police officer, you can learn a great deal from research into the types of incidents that lead to shootings as well as the types of incidents (and all the dynamics involved) that lead to police officers being killed.

Private citizens can also learn from these events, but they can learn even more from listening to news stories about crime victims. Why were these victims targeted? Where did the confrontation occur? What were the victims doing at the time? And, most importantly, what did they do that marked them as targets? What were the criminal's tactics? How was he armed? What are the typical dynamics of confrontations with criminals? Learn these things and expect that your opponent will be a well-prepared, physically strong, and motivated criminal warrior. Prepare to defeat him and not the emaciated drug-addict with a dull pocketknife, and you will probably do well. Understanding the nature of your opponent, as well as the attitudes of victims, will be invaluable in minimizing another uncertainty: that of the outcome of battle. This knowledge will help more than that new custom blaster, that new video on knife drills, or that

Introduction

high-dollar course at the new Middle Eastern Hostage Rescue Gunfighting Academy.

Along with knowing as much about your opponent as possible, you must have an honest understanding of your own abilities and, more importantly, attitude. The mythical police hero Dirty Harry once said, "A man has to know his limitations." There are all sorts of self-created pompous fools, with their wannabe chests full of self-issued medals, who "think they can" but in fact can't and never will. A wise warrior knows his limits, and while he tries to extend them, when it's for real he always operates within them.

The most important part of this self-evaluation of ability is honesty. You can lie to your girlfriend(s) about how accurate you are, you can lie to your partners about how fast you are, and you can even lie to the criminals about your willingness to do them in. But whatever you do, never, ever lie to yourself about what you can do or are prepared to do. Uncertainty about yourself or your skills will kill you just as easily as a slash to your jugular.

As we will see, the right mental attitude has an extraordinary effect on the outcome of battle. But what about fate? We really cannot develop an intel file on what will happen, but we can certainly plot the possibilities, much like a flow chart. What are the possibilities in a fight?

You can win or lose. We already discussed the possibilities of winning. What if you lose? What if you are killed? What will happen to your family and loved

The Combative Perspective

ones? Boy, talk about uncertainties! As much as it brings disquiet, to be truly comfortable in this environment, you must understand and accept the possibility of your death. No one wants to die, but only a fool never thinks about it. It is important that while you do everything to avoid it, you accept this possibility. It's important that you have a clear mind when the final exam is placed in front of you.

Be certain that you have sufficient medical coverage so that you are sure to get any required medical treatment after a fight. Injuries often take many months, if not years, to heal. Injured and alive is better than dead, but getting back to full strength will take time and care. Buy life insurance so that your family will be cared for after your death. Don't put off things that you know you'd regret not having done if you were killed in a fight tomorrow. Strive to minimize, if not eliminate, this source of uncertainty as well.

Having eliminated uncertainty and hesitation, the next step is to avoid surprise by cultivating a level of watchfulness and awareness that will provide an early warning signal of an impending confrontation. This will be discussed at length in Part Three.

Once you have cultivated a desire to win, eliminated uncertainty, and developed a state of mind where you are attentive to your environment and aware of your situation, there remains only one thing. That final element of the combative perspective is by far the most important of all, without which everything else is moot. That, my friends, is willingness. Without the deliberate

INTRODUCTION

will to harm those "fellow human beings" who would choose you as prey, all of the training, study, and attentiveness on earth will not help you. Willingness is, again, one of those things that cannot be learned but rather must be developed by the individual.

I will attempt to dissect all of the elements of the combative perspective and present them to you in a logical and scientific manner. I hope that the end result will be the peace of mind that comes from preparedness, understanding, and strength.

DESIRE FOR VICTORY

Part One

I know an officer who was once bushwacked by a much larger and stronger adversary one night. After ten seconds into the very one-sided fight, Phil had several broken ribs, a dislocated shoulder, an ear that hung by a strip of skin, and enough asphalt rash to qualify for a Bactine commercial. Yet, as he lay on the deck and felt his enemy's hand reach for the holstered SIG by his side, a primal, meat-eating rage rose within him. Phil ignored his injuries and exploded toward his enemy, turning the tables on him and so soundly

The Combative Perspective

beating him that only the responding units saved the criminal's life by intervening. For Phil, what made the difference between life and death was something you could never teach in a police academy, martial arts dojo, or civilian concealed carry weapon (CCW) class. More than the desire to win, and far beyond the "never give in" doctrine, we are talking about <u>the desire to destroy your attacker.</u> This desire must be harnessed and controlled, and never allowed to run away from you, but <u>it is necessary nonetheless.</u> Call it controlled rage, call it whatever you want, but it is a focused and channeled desire to close with and destroy those who would hurt you. Theodore Roosevelt wrote about "the power of joy in battle" when he referred to "<u>the wolf rising in the heart.</u>" This is powerful stuff from another age that is nevertheless essential in our modern world.

Chapter 1

What Desire Is Made Of

My organization, Suarez International Training Group, conducts a handful of instructor development courses every year. The attendees range from private industry trainers to professional military men to police officer/rangemasters. Invariably, one of the most often heard questions is, "How do I motivate my students?"

It seems that in some areas, notably in modern law enforcement, there is a tangible lack of motivation, or desire, on the part of many students. A lack of desire to excel in the study of arms eventually leads to the lack of desire to win a fight. Although technical proficiency is an important part of the puzzle, winning a fight is more a matter of the level of desire than of technical proficiency.

The Combative Perspective

The desire to win comprises several factors: knowledge of existing ability, acceptance of the possibility of Injury, purity and intensity of focus, and the perception that there are no alternatives.

KNOWLEDGE OF EXISTING ABILITY

Most students (of the gun, the knife, or unarmed combatives) spend the bulk of their time developing and establishing the knowledge of existing ability. This is important because if you are not sure you can win the fight there will be a great deal of hesitation, and thus a lack of desire. To quote the patron saint of rogue cops, "A man has to know his limitations." Likewise, it's handy to know what you actually can do on demand. From ability comes confidence. Confidence minimizes fear and apprehension. And that is essential to the birth of the desire to win.

ACCEPTANCE OF THE POSSIBILITY OF INJURY

It's been said that if you get into a knife fight, you will be cut, or if you get into a gunfight, you will be shot. This is not necessarily true, as many men (myself included) have been in both without suffering cuts or gunshot wounds. Nevertheless, the possibility of injury or even death is very real. Fear of death or injury is part of our psyche, yet it can be overcome. (If you overcome the fear of death, overcoming fear of injury is a no-brainer.) The question, of course, is *how?* There is no book to read or class to attend to reach this level. It's a spiritual issue that each individual must come to terms with.

PURITY AND INTENSITY OF FOCUS

When I teach a pistol course, we spend a great deal of time on visual verification via the sights. We discuss the need to visually focus on the front sight so that the target and the rear sight may be kept in alignment with the front sight, and thus the shot will go where it is intended. We point out that since the human eye can only focus on one specific distance, or point, it's best to focus on the front sight. The results bear out the theory.

The human mind is very much like the human eye. It cannot, under the stress of combat, focus on more than one thought or idea. Rather than try to fight this, we must embrace it as a strength.

Developing intensity and purity of focus will make you a better fighter. Success in fighting, as we mentioned before, is more a matter of attitude than anything else. The ability to mentally focus intensely and exclusively for short periods of time is an important skill. It is nothing "spooky" or new age, or anything of the sort. It is simply the human mind working at peak performance and the well-trained body obeying its commands.

One practice that I've found very useful for developing this mental ability is heavy weight lifting. I've found

The Combative Perspective

that the level of mental focus evident when handling very heavy (near maximum level) weight is the same as that necessary in a fight. I'm discussing powerlifting-type exertion, not the 25 sets of 25 repetitions of a spandex-clad body sculptor. There are other methods as well, such as short-distance sprinting or swimming, wrestling and other combatives, etc. The advantage of weight training is that it can be done alone.

Purity and intensity of focus will allow you to exclude other distractions, such as emotional over-reaction to danger, as well as fear and fright.

I was once questioned by a squeamish admin-type SWAT commander (the kind that sits in an office all day wearing black BDUs, tactical nylon, and velcro) if I was afraid during the gunfight in question. My honest response was that I was too busy winning the fight to worry about whether I was supposed to be afraid or not. Intense purity of focus!

THE PERCEPTION THAT THERE ARE NO ALTERNATIVES

In our modern, veggie-eating world, we are taught to believe that there are always alternatives to violence. Sometimes there are not. In a fight, sometimes the only alternative to defeat and death is to win by destroying your adversary. This is clear to the man who stands his ground in the hallway of his home facing three armed invaders, with his wife and infant children behind him. Its also clear to the police officer who is knocked to the

What Desire Is Made Of

ground and then feels hands grabbing for his holstered gun. And let's not forget the soldier who, separated from his unit, finds himself surrounded by the enemy—one that is not known for fair treatment of prisoners.

The perception that there is no way out other than to overcome is a powerful realization and a powerful tool. Often there *are* ways out . . . before the fight is joined. But once the first shot is fired or the first blade is drawn, the desire to win will often decide the outcome. The desire to win will allow you ignore broken bones or injuries that would cause most others to shrink away. The desire to win will allow you to focus on winning the fight to the exclusion of distracting thoughts about your own self-preservation. In the end, the desire to win, when mixed with the ability to win, will help you do just that.

ELIMINATION OF UNCERTAINTY

Part Two

Who doesn't remember Val Kilmer's classic line in *Tombstone* as he (playing Doc Holliday) faced an impending gun duel against the reputed gunman Johnny Ringo? Doc smiled and told Johnny Ringo, "Say when."

One of the things I've learned about people facing a fight is that they experience a great deal of uncertainty about when the line is actually crossed, that is, when the red flag really has gone up. It's almost as if they are asking someone to follow them around and "say when" they are legally able to unleash violence upon an aggressor. The main concern of many people is just exactly when are they are safe,

The Combative Perspective

legally speaking, in blasting the bejeebers out of some miscreant.

There are other uncertainties. There is often uncertainty about nature and intent of the adversary. If you do not believe that there are bad people out there who intend to do you and/or your loved ones harm, then you will not be mentally prepared to do what is necessary to defend your lives when faced with a hostile aggressor. However, statistics and experience do not lie, and there are plenty of both out there to demonstrate in no uncertain terms that not only do these evildoers exist, but they will not hesitate to take your life if you give them an opening.

The outcome of the fight is another unknown that can cause a great deal of trepidation. Even with all the tactical training in the world, there is no way of knowing for certain how your skills and abilities are going to stack up against those of your enemy.

In reality, there are three possible outcomes: We may die in the fight. We may die in the fight as we ourselves kill our attacker. Or—the only good outcome—we may kill our adversary and remain unharmed.

Although we will leave this topic for another book, a warrior must accept the possibility of his own death. That is not to say that one needs an extreme embracing of death, as is found in some Asian cultures. But a modern fighter must nevertheless accept the possibility, and moreover, he must be comfortable with it.

Skill and ability aside, there is a great deal of evidence to suggest that the attitude of the person under attack has an overwhelming impact on the outcome of the battle. As you will see, adopting the right mental attitude can go a long way toward eliminating any uncertainty about the outcome or whether you will be a victim or a victor in the fight of your life.

Chapter 2

LIABILITY

The uncertainty surrounding civil and or criminal liability is a major concern for most people involved in the study of defensecraft. Some are more afraid of this possibility than they are about the actual gunfight. The reason, I think, is that most students believe they can control—or at least affect—the outcome of a fight. They don't feel the same about the untamed wild animal known as the legal system. They view this as some sort of mysterious monster that will come in the night and devour them, their bank account, and their home in the wink of a politician's eye.

Keying in on this fear, stories abound in the defensecraft community. Almost every day someone repeats some horror story he or she heard at the gun

The Combative Perspective

store or the dojo. Invariably, it involves a well-meaning homeowner or business owner who was forced to defend himself against some hideous career barbarian. The hero of the story usually flattens his attacker masterfully, killing or wounding him, only to be hauled into court afterward, stripped of all his worldly possessions, given 40 lashes, and sentenced to a lengthy prison term. Such stories, like most legends, are usually exaggerated beyond any credibility but are widely accepted and believed by a community that rightfully fears the courtroom.

Some of the problem also comes from the law enforcement community. A police officer has a much greater chance of being sued than any private citizen. The badge is not a symbol of honor or trust from the community. No, friends, the badge is simply a big, bright target (it's in the fine print of the contract). After a confrontation with a police officer is over, the survivor (or his surviving relatives) will often try to stick his grubby little paws into the deep pockets of the agency involved. Lawsuits affect the city's political machine, and, therefore, they affect the office of the chief of police. Consequently, since smelly stuff rolls downhill, policies are crafted in order to insulate agencies and administrators, as much as possible, from litigation.

The line troops are now so browbeaten by their chiefs about this stuff that the fear of a lawsuit shrinks many departments into impotent, ineffective agencies, afraid of the very criminals they are supposed to confront. When civilian friends approach these officers for advice about liability issues surrounding self-defense, you can well imagine the picture the officers paint. Death before litigation is the overriding feeling.

The literary community and media don't help the situation at all. Many well-intentioned (and some not-so-well-intentioned) writers fan the flames of fear by penning articles and books that effectively convey the message that it's better to be killed than sued! Most of these authors are not attorneys, and they have never had to "face death in the alley," much less criminal or civil legal proceedings from the seat of "defendant." They are simply repeating the same stories and propagating the same fears that routinely circulate in the defensecraft community. I suspect they would not sell many books if they all wrote, "Everything will be fine."

I can't help but think that in repeating these horror stories, the fear mongers conveniently leave out critical details. The heroic figure that was sentenced to 10 years in jail for winning a gunfight likely had a few other little things going on in his situation. Did he have to kill his attacker in his home or business, or was it outside Demon Joe's Skull and Bones Biker Bar at 0300 after a couple of six-packs of Corona? Was his attacker a total stranger, or was it his former business partner who is now dating his ex-wife? Was the winner of the fight a respected person in the community and the evil attacker a stunt double for Hannibal the

The Combative Perspective

Cannibal, or was it the other way around? Do these types of possibilities change the picture a little bit? Sure they do. All of these little side issues that really have nothing to do with an incident tactically will have a great bearing when the event is examined in a courtroom. Generally speaking, if you acted correctly, you will probably be all right. If you were not legal in carrying or possessing your weapon, or if you should not have been at that place and at that time when the fight began, it will be questioned. Your answers to questions concerning your conduct will determine your future.

Bear in mind that the burden of proof relative to self-defense is generally on the prosecution. That means that the prosecution must prove beyond a reasonable doubt that you did not act in self-defense, rather than your having to prove you did. Unless there are other issues, the prosecution's case is extremely difficult to make. They may try if you are an unpopular sort, but it's all uphill for them.

In reality, while everything might not exactly be fine in the aftermath of your defending your life in a fight, neither will it be as horrible as they paint it. Might there be civil repercussions if you shoot an adversary in a gunfight? Sure, it's possible. Might you face some sort of criminal prosecution if you kill an armed criminal with a knife or other weapon? Again, the possibility is there. But remember also that you may very well be killed if you don't take care of business when the evil ones come to test you.

LIABILITY

SAY "WHEN"—THE RULES OF ENGAGEMENT

Lawful self-defense is always a complete defense to a charged crime. This is difficult to address fully in a book, since readers may be located in areas with completely different laws. Nevertheless, survival takes precedence over *any* laws, and that usually means that you must win. It's sort of the old "judged or carried" thing, but within reason. I strongly suggest becoming intimately familiar with the laws on this matter in the state and city where you live. The following guidelines, however, should cover most civilized parts of the world. If the place where you reside does not allow you to fight to save your life, again, my only suggestion is *move*.

Generally speaking, you have the right to use deadly force in self-defense under certain circumstances. However, one thing that must be present is your full understanding of the rules of engagement under which you operate. The core defensive concept of most police use-of-force policies, as well as guidelines for civilians, is Immediate Defense of Life (IDOL).

Perception of Threat

First and foremost, you must honestly and reasonably believe you were in danger of being killed, seriously injured, or sexually assaulted and be able to explain why. This means the belief must be seen legally as both honest and reasonable. However, your belief need not be correct. In other words, if you *believed*

The Combative Perspective

you were in such danger, and that belief was reasonable, you are *not* criminally liable, even if you were incorrect in your perceptions.

For example, suppose you are walking in a rough part of town when some night creature aggressively jumps out of the darkness toward you, brandishing a long cylindrical object that you would bet the farm is a long-barreled revolver. So you blast him to smithereens, fully convinced he was about to kill you with his eight-inch-barreled S&W 686. Only it turns out he was a street psycho with a fireplace lighting tool! Bad situation, but you acted legally based on your perceptions, beliefs, and state of mind. (By the way, this one really happened, and the shooter was not charged.)

The right to defend others is essentially the same as the right to defend yourself. If you're acting against a group, self-defense can be claimed as a legal defense when deadly force is used against any member of the group who was perceived to have threatened death or serious injury. However, you can't attack all of them because they were standing in the same corner when their companion tried to rob you. There must be more to it than that.

Amount of Force

In addition, the amount of force must be consistent with the threat. You can't use deadly force to combat a threat of minor injury (e.g., a punch in the nose). There is a corollary to this rule about disparity of force: If the

LIABILITY

aggressor of the "punch in the nose" is a steroid-abusing Visigoth in his 20s and you are a frail 90-year-old, you can assume that a punch in the face by someone like him will be a very serious life-altering threat indeed. You are therefore justified in using deadly force, based on the amount of damage he is likely to cause you. The same defense is not available to you, however, if you are a 200-pound power-lifting kickboxing champion in the same situation.

The legal requirement that the use of self-defense must be reasonable has direct implications for the trained tactical shooter. What is a reasonable response for a person with no training will not be deemed reasonable for a SWAT point man, an ex-GSG9 commando, or a multiple graduate of our flourishing modern-day Salles de Armes.

A trained person will be expected to know the difference between a minor threat and a life-threatening assault. A trained person might also be expected to resolve the matter with less force (greater accuracy and less violence) than would a neophyte (for whom panic may be excusable). If you are a high-speed/low-drag type, hold your standards high, because everyone else will do the same.

One issue that draws a great deal of concern here is that of equipment. We've all seen the articles—"Custom Guns Will Kill You in Court," "The Liability-Free Martial Art," "The Lawyer-Proof Bowie Knife," ad nauseum.

I had one student come to a course with a pistol that had been court-proofed to such a degree that it

The Combative Perspective

was totally useless as a fighting tool. The poor fellow would have been better off hitting an attacker on the head with it than actually trying to shoot him.

Will the gun you use create a civil or criminal liability problem for you? In some cases it might, but in most cases it will not. What are some things that *will* increase the liability potential for you? How about using an illegal weapon? That will certainly do it! Although you may disagree with many of the asinine gun laws that pass the desks of our silly legislators, when it comes to working weapons, you must make sure you are super legal. This certainly means your personal blaster should be registered to you, and all the paperwork (including carry permits) should be current. This can also mean avoiding weapons that might be labeled "assault weapons." Shoot the intruder with a 30-30 lever-action rifle, and not with that Galil .223 Israeli assault rifle. Use your Remington 870, and not the streetsweeper. Defend yourself with the benign Trailmaster and not the evil-sounding custom Navy SEAL attack knife. You get the idea. The impact you make on your adversary will feel the same to him regardless of which weapon actually did the damage.

How about light triggers, special sights, and all of those other things we use to customize our personal weapons to help us use them better? These will only become issues if you make a mistake and either miss or shoot the wrong person. If additions or improvements to your weapon help you hit more quickly and accurately, then use them, as long as the weapon's reliability is not adversely affected. Just be sure that that you or your attorney can offer a reasonable, articulate explanation in court as to why you added these accessories to your gun. Much the same applies to ammunition selection and so forth.

Are there cases where such issues might have caused legal problems? Sure there are, but there are exceptions to every rule. The bottom line is, if you are going to try to make a weapon completely liability free, you might as well unload it, put it in the safe, and never carry it.

What about readers who do not rely on firearms but on edged weapons or a variety of other weapons or martial arts skills? Pretty much the same principles apply. Don't think that you won't be scrutinized in court because you killed the guy with a karate chop instead of an AK-47. Dead is still dead, and skill is still skill.

Immediacy of Threat

Finally, the danger must be perceived as immediate. A threat to do harm in the future does not legally justify self-defense. You cannot cut someone's head off for promising that "one day" he will kill you and your whole family. There are other ways to deal with this threat, but immediate deadly force is not one of them.

In some locations, a person must try to retreat before using deadly force if it is safe to do so. This is a tactically foolish law, obviously penned by those who have no understanding about how these things are. If you run, the adversary will often chase you. Thankfully,

The Combative Perspective

this law does not generally apply in one's own home. Just remember your situation and keep that in mind. Retreat only to the point where it would place you in tactical jeopardy, then stand and fight like a monster!

The Bottom Line

According to the IDOL standard, when faced with a tactical problem requiring a deadly-force decision, you (civilian, police officer, or whatever) must ask yourself the question, "If I don't stop this man, right now, will he seriously injure or kill someone?" If the answer is no, or if there is any doubt, then immediate violence on your part is not the answer. The pure reason of this concept cannot be disputed.

I hope I've answered the question of when "legally." When "tactically" may be little different.

I received a call one day from an acquaintance from Europe. This man is one of those ultra-marathoners who eats tofu and grains and runs 20 miles a day while listening to Zen rock. He'd been to a course with me on the Continent and knew that I frequented the desert regions from time to time. He was intent on spending his vacation running across Death Valley! After I questioned his sanity a few times, he assured me that it was not going to be a problem. He was, however, concerned about the wildlife—more specifically, rattlesnakes. They don't have them in his part of the world, and he wanted to know how he could tell one when he saw it. I told him he'd know when he saw one.

The same goes for knowing that an aggressor means business. *You'll know.* First impressions are usually correct. Don't dismiss them. There will be the obvious clues (gun in hand, raised machete, etc.), and there will be some other not-so-obvious clues. Don't try to rationalize them away. Instead, pay attention to them! They are saying "WHEN."

In wrestling with the question of when it is appropriate to use lethal force in defending your life, the concern over criminal and civil repercussions must not be your primary focus. *Winning the fight takes precedence.* There are no appeals from the grave. In a worst-case scenario where you are both sued and imprisoned, you can always regain your freedom and rebuild your fortune. But it's unlikely that anyone will be able to breathe life back into your slashed up, broken, or bullet-riddled but liability-free corpse as the flies collect around you on the pavement! Lawsuits are a bad thing, yes. But so are funerals. Especially if you're the guest of honor.

AFTER-ACTION PROCEDURES

So let's assume for a moment that you have just fought for your life and won. Everything you did was tactically correct. All of the time and money spent training paid off tonight when the serial rapist you'd heard about on the evening news picked your house as his target. It was a fatal choice. He is lying face down in your living room, and the air is thick with the smell of gun smoke.

THE COMBATIVE PERSPECTIVE

You notice, in one of those strange, detached moments that are common in battle, how perfectly symmetrical the growing bloodstain appears in the tan Berber carpeting. Your wife's hysterical scream jolts you back into reality.

Not a pleasant story to contemplate . . . having to replace that rug and all.

In all seriousness, I've just described the ending of a fight. This *should* be the end of it: You, the good guy, have killed the bad guy. End of story! But in our mixed-up and strange society, there are those who might want to make more of it than that. And so, the reality is that this could be the beginning of another fight.

Notice that I said *could*, and not *shall*. Again, there is no guarantee that you will face any administrative, criminal, or civil problems after winning a fight. However, you never really know. So, in the interest of preparedness, let's give some thought to insulating ourselves from these after-the-fact problems.

Again, winning the fight takes top billing on the tactical "to-do" list. But there are some other things that need to be seen to immediately afterwards. Primarily, your goal is to cover yourself with the "mantle of innocence" so that if things get sticky later you will have something to point to and say, "See, that's what a good guy would do."

First thing is to see to yourself and your protectees. Are you or any of your protectees (family members) injured? If so, medical attention for them (or you) is paramount. As far as I'm concerned, that piece of you-

LIABILITY

know-what can bleed to death right there on the Berber rug while you deal with any victims.

Second thing is to calm down. You will be excited. Boy, will you be excited! Calm down. Calm your family down. You should have briefed them on exactly what to do and what not to do in such a case. Regardless, they will be very agitated. Get everyone on board as far as mental and emotional control. If there are little ones involved, then it's up to you to set the example. The last thing you need at the moment is to have hysterical family members clouding your thoughts.

Third thing, call the police. Some have suggested calling your attorney first, but this may be viewed as consciousness of guilt, especially if the bad guy died due to lack of medical care, which he theoretically could have received if you had called the police first. You should know ahead of time exactly what you are going to say. Remember, it's all recorded. Understand also that the responding officers only know what they've been told. Begin forming the correct impression in their minds with what you tell the dispatcher.

If you say something like, "There's a dead guy on my rug, and I'm not saying anything else until I talk to my mouthpiece," you will be treated and perceived a certain way. The goal is to let the officers know that there has been a self-defense shooting and that you are the victim. Here's a suggested method:

> Hello, do you have my address on your 911 screen? [If they do not, give it to them.] I am a

The Combative Perspective

victim of a crime. There's been a shooting. The aggressor is down and needs an ambulance. Please send help.

In this brief exchange, you've colored yourself as the good-guy victim and the dead guy as the bad-guy home invader. You have not said anything that you'll regret later. They may ask you pertinent tactical questions such as, "Did you shoot him," "How many bad guys are there," and so on. All I can suggest here is that you not be deceitful. You can answer things such as would be pertinent to responding officers. If there is anything that you do not want recorded, simply tell the dispatcher that you'll talk to the officers when they arrive. Give the dispatcher your description, and remind him or her that you are the victim.

When the officers arrive, do not have your weapon in hand! Have it secured, either on your person or elsewhere, but not in your hand. The officers will have a brief picture in their minds about what happened based on what the dispatcher told them. They are naturally skeptical due to their experience, and although they will have formed opinions based on the call, they will make up their own minds when they arrive.

Some suggestions: Even though this portion of things will be lengthy and tiresome, be as cooperative as you can without giving up any rights. If you are uncomfortable with anything they are asking, object to it. Generally, the truth of the matter will be evident, and they will probably act accordingly.

LIABILITY

They may be a little rough initially. Understand that all they know is that there has been a shooting. Allow them to take control of the scene, and allow the initial tension to diffuse itself. If they ask you for your weapon, do not just grab it and bring it out. Be very slow about this, and ask them how they'd like you to obtain it. You may even want to point to it and have them take possession of it themselves. Understand that the weapon will be taken as evidence for a while. It's not special treatment for you; that's just the way it's done. If they ask about other weapons in the house, that's an area that is not pertinent to the investigation and is none of their business.

How about what to say when they ask that famous question, "What happened?" There are three possibilities here: 1) tell them everything because you are a certified Good Guy and have absolutely nothing to hide, 2) don't say a darned thing, and 3) give a brief story establishing what took place and then ask to see your attorney.

If you believe number one is the best option, you also probably use *Adam-12* and *Kung Fu* reruns as training films! Even (perhaps especially) police officers mistrust their own agencies when they've been involved in shootings. Spilling your guts is never a good idea, even if you really have nothing to hide.

The "Say Nothing" school of thought is preferable to the "Tell 'Em Everything" philosophy. However, the former is not adopted without a price. Police administrators will often tell you that their investigations are

The Combative Perspective

always fair and impartial. That is the biggest lie since the free democracy. Their investigations are colored by their perspectives and impressions as to what they've seen, or sometimes (for some) by what they want to see. If officers roll up to a homicide and the only live guy there isn't talking, the case will probably be handled like a murder. Bottom line is that we don't know what happened, the dead guy can't give us anything, and the live guy is not talking. We will not leave that scene empty-handed. Even your attorney will not be able to redirect the investigation once it's begun.

I have a suggestion of compromises. First, understand that I am not an attorney and I am not giving you legal advice. I have, however, been on that end of things several times in my career. It is upon that empirical experience that I base my suggestions.

I advocate making a brief (very brief) noncommittal statement to the officers and then asking to speak with your attorney. Something like this:

> Officers, this man broke into my house [point to the broken front door], threatened to kill me and my family [point to six diapered kids huddling around their mother in the far corner], and I had to protect them. Now gentlemen, I have never had anything like this happen to me. I'd like to see to my family and call my attorney before I say anything else.

And then don't say anything else until you have

LIABILITY

your backup there with you. Oh, by the way, don't call your buddy the paralegal or your corporate attorney. Develop an acquaintance with a bona fide criminal attorney (preferably, one who is in the business of protecting police officers in shootings), and call him!

Another point you must know is that the police profession is populated with good guys as well as devilish, backstabbing, politically aspiring, certifiable bad guys. You never know who you will get. Some officers in the latter category will try to trick you or be sneaky about violating your rights. Be careful, and be alert.

Also, if you have any sort of medical problems or are experiencing chest pains or other such symptoms, you need to have a doctor examine you immediately. The potential stress of a fight to the finish affects everyone differently. If your system is already physically weak and you begin to feel symptoms, pay attention to them. No agency will allow any of its officers to interrogate anyone in such a condition. Few chiefs want a citizen going flat-line with a heart attack during an interview. Make certain that family members are also briefed about this stuff.

OK, I hope I haven't scared the willies out of you with all of this. This chapter was intended, above all, to temper your anxiety surrounding the idea that the end of one fight *could be* the beginning of another one.

In general, if you acted properly, everything will be all right.

Chapter 3

The Nature and Intent of the Adversary

Sometimes the beginning of the battle will be easy to recognize. This is not always the case, however. Sometimes there may be indecision and rationalization on your part about what is actually happening. When you are facing these "grey battles," the only thing that will give you a headstart will be a study of just who your potential adversary may be and what he has in mind.

In this amazing age of information, rare is the person with an interest in tactics and personal defense who has not heard of the FBI Uniform Crime Report. This lengthy document lists statistics obtained from throughout the United States on a variety of subjects related to crime. Going back several years, these statistics tell a tale of trends in urban combat. The reports

The Combative Perspective

are quite lengthy, and there have not been many dramatic changes through the years, so I will not spend a great deal of time on a year-by-year analysis. Officers and civilians alike can learn from the information available in the Uniform Crime Report. Additionally, the report has served as a guide for trainers and students of defensecraft in organizing their training.

Of specific importance to those in law enforcement has always been the section of the report dealing with police officers killed. There are a number of reasons for this, primary among them being the fact that nobody wants to get killed. By learning how our brothers and sisters fell, law enforcement officers can hope to avoid similar events. Unfortunately, there is a negative slant to the report in that it lists only failures. It would be nice if there were a set of statistics on "armed criminals killed by police," but apparently such things are not available. In our society, the winners tend to keep quiet about it. Nevertheless, we can learn many things from the statistics that this report does make available.

In short, these reports show that urban fights (with guns or otherwise) involving police officers tend to be close range, high-intensity events characterized by sudden violence. There are often more bad guys than there are good guys, and the light levels are generally not that good. Since these fights tend to be short in duration, the number of effective shots fired, or hits delivered, is minimal (there is usually no time for more before the issue is decided).

The Nature and Intent of the Adversary

Nothing is new there, but the areas dealing with attackers yield some invaluable information that is often ignored. Although it is dangerous to categorize our adversaries (you may meet one who doesn't fit the mold), the statistics can tell us a great deal about them and their motivations and intent.

This may be controversial stuff in our age of "kinder, gentler policing," but all I'm concerned about is keeping the good guys alive. Political and social issues are beneath my interests. Social trends are what they are, and it's not our job in this context to fix them, only to understand them.

Most of the criminals who killed a police officer had begun their criminal careers around the tender age of 12. Furthermore, 48 percent of those interviewed stated that they had killed, or at least tried to kill, another man prior to their confrontation with the officers. (This statistic includes incidents involving knives, physical force, and guns.) A much higher percentage of cop killers admitted to other crimes of violence (lesser crimes than murder or attempted murder). In addition, 74 percent admitted to carrying a firearm or other weapon at all times (so much for laws being a deterrent), and 54 percent admitted to practicing with their weapons at least once a month (just what sort of practice we don't know).

A high percentage of those who had killed a police officer had been cut, shot, or fired upon at some point in their lives. When asked about this, the overwhelming attitude was that they did not intend to allow anyone to

43

The Combative Perspective

ever shoot them again and would shoot first to prevent it. Moreover, their generally aggressive attitude included the belief that they had the tactical advantage over police officers because *they already knew what they would do.*

So your job is to take this intelligence we've gathered on your potential adversary and begin formulating a series of possible plans based on where you might encounter him.

Of even greater significance is the information available on the victims in these gunfights, and the next chapter will address that topic at length. Now, I must point out that it would never be proper to talk ill of the fallen good guys who've paid the ultimate price. But at the same time, we must learn from these events and the lessons they hold. The goal here is to save the lives of the good guys (the bad guys' contributions to the culture we can do without). Again, we are seeking not to denigrate or criticize these victims but to learn from their unfortunate circumstances.

Chapter 4

VICTIM OR VICTOR?
ATTITUDE IS EVERYTHING

The statistical data presented in the previous chapter should leave no shadow of doubt regarding the mind-set of the criminal aggressor. But even when people understand in no uncertain terms that the intent of these predators is to kill them, many still wrestle with doubts about their own skills and abilities and uncertainty as to how they will fare in a fight for their lives. But in determining the outcome of such a fight, skill is only part of the picture.

When it comes to behavioral descriptors of victims, be they police officers or civilians, statistical research and empirical evidence point to some interesting differences between victims and criminals. This information can teach us a great deal about the role attitude plays in either making us look like easy prey or like someone to

The Combative Perspective

avoid. When you are wrestling with uncertainty, it is reassuring to know that attitude is often the determining factor in the outcome of a fight.

FALLEN GOOD GUYS

The following descriptors for police officers killed in gunfights were obtained from open-ended questions in interviews of the victims' peers and supervisors. These same questions were used, when possible, in interviewing suspects who knew the victim officers prior to the event. Including these diverse perspectives helped to avoid the situation where only good things would be said by the officers' associates.

Suspects and colleagues alike characterized the victim-officer as someone who is friendly to everyone, tends to use less force than other officers and is often reluctant to use force, tends to perceive his or her role as more public relations than law enforcement, does not follow sound tactical guidelines (i.e., takes shortcuts), tends to look for "good" in others, and is laid back and easygoing. Significantly, 57 percent of the criminals interviewed described the victim as unprepared.

Together with the statistical data presented in the previous chapter, these findings paint a picture of an unsuspecting, slow-to-violence Officer Friendly being stalked by an evil predator who has already made up his mind to do violence. (The tragedy is that in the modern police profession such an officer is the overwhelming choice of the brass, both as a recruit and for career advancement.)

The lesson here is that attitude and the silent signals it sends will either mark you as a hard target to be avoided at all costs or as easy prey. Unfortunately, the former might also mark you for frivolous personnel complaints that many agencies accept routinely. I've always had a difficult time concealing my attitude toward the bad guys and have sometimes suffered the "slings and arrows" of headhunting politicians as a result. It is a Catch 22—don't be too friendly and easygoing, but don't look too mean, lest you get called in to talk to the city manager.

The bottom line is that there are evil people out there. They've always been out there, and no amount of social engineering, community policing, or legislation against freedom will ever change that. In order to fight evil people, you need good people, fully capable of controlled preemptive or retaliatory violence, to stand against them. You do not need, nor will you be effective with, an army of highly educated but squeamish, weak-willed social workers or bureaucratic cheerleaders in uniform. *There is no nice, clean, or politically correct way to deal with an armed and violent predator who has no intention of being dealt with.*

So where does that leave today's officers? Their job is more difficult now than ever because not only do they have to be tigers, but also they have to keep their hunger for meat hidden under "sheep's clothing."

To stay alive in order to enjoy retirement, they must remember that the evil ones do not have their same val-

The Combative Perspective

ues, nor do they give a rodent's posterior what the department's mission statement is. These evil ones will try to kill them with absolutely no regard for use-of-force policies, IA investigations, or newspaper articles. In order to win, officers must be able to respond reflexively with a level of violence greater than that offered by their adversaries. They must be trained and taught that although they may need to have a shiny veneer of community orientation, when the time comes to face the evil ones, the same tactics will be used as have always been used. Sudden violence is only overcome with greater violence.

Strong words? Perhaps, but as I said, my interest is in showing you, the reader, the essentials of winning the fight, as ugly as they may be. I suppose I'm sort of passionate about this stuff. There are plenty of noble things to die for, but some administrative numbskull's idea of political propriety is not one of them. Remember, winning the fight is the only option. When you lose, you'll probably die. Even if you had to use "brutal" means that get you fired, you're still alive to get another job.

FIGHT DYNAMICS FOR CIVILIANS

I know of no statistical data similar in nature to the FBI Uniform Crime Report relating to citizen (nonpolice) fights. No exhaustive study has been done of citizens who win confrontations against bad guys. Such a set of stats, if it existed, would also undoubtedly include innumerable cases of the "good riddance" fac-

Victim or Victor? Attitude Is Everything

tor (bad guy vs. bad guy). We can examine standard crime data to learn about times, dates, types of crime, and so on, but that doesn't tell us much more than the method of victimization.

Lack of official statistics notwithstanding, I have had the opportunity to be first-responder as well as investigator in a number of cases that typify citizen fights. In some, the citizen was suitably prepared and routed the criminals. In others, the reverse was true; an unprepared citizen met his fate at the hands of his attackers.

Let's examine a few real-life scenarios to see how critical a factor attitude can be in determining the outcome of such a fight.

* * *

Case #1—Unarmed and unprepared emergency room technician (who shared many of the victim officers' behavioral descriptors) came home late at night and left his keys in the front door lock. Now, bear in mind that this man was an extremely strong power lifter.

A trio of predatory hoodlums entered his home and roused him from sleep. Even though he clearly outmatched them in size and strength, and even though they were unarmed, the victim surrendered. They hogtied him on his kitchen floor with a lamp cord and proceeded to ransack his home. After filling their pockets with what they could find, they stomped him to death right by his Westinghouse dishwasher.

Attitude?

The Combative Perspective

* * *

Case #2—Jewelry salesman arrived home after a gem show. As he pulled into his underground garage, he noticed two figures slip into the garage in the darkness. He was aware of this being a potential weakness in his habits, and although he hadn't changed his procedures, he always kept alert at these times.

He palmed the 1911 .45-caliber pistol that he always carried with him, threw the transmission into park, and quickly got out of his car. He saw two males sporting ski masks approaching him. One held a CZ-75 pistol and the other a Lorcin .380. Not waiting for the inevitable discussion regarding property rights, he fired.

Although his marksmanship was insufficient, his courage was not. The crooks dropped their weapons and ran for the hills. We found a blood trail where one of his rounds had undoubtedly nicked the hoodlum, but to this day, no body (I mean no one) ever turned up.

The would-be victim was treated to a hearty handshake and a pat on the back by yours truly. No charges were filed, and after the investigation was completed his .45 was returned to him.

Attitude!

* * *

Case #3—Hoodlum with an axe broke into a high-dollar home while the residents were there. After

Victim or Victor? Attitude Is Everything

announcing that he was planning on killing everyone in sight, he began his best award-winning imitation of Jack Nicholson in *The Shining*.

The peaceful man of the house, lacking any weapon with which to fight, and being on the low-testosterone side of the charts, was last seen running away . . . leaving his wife and baby behind!

The wife, apparently more of a man than he was, tried to escape with her child in hand. She was met at the front door by Jack Nicholson's stunt double, who embedded the axe between her shoulder blades in the best Viking tradition and then tried to test the Solomon concept on the child. She lived, after an embarrassingly nonviolent police response, but neither she nor her child will ever be the same.

This unfortunate family hated weapons and refused to have them in their home. They hadn't got the word that unarmed men can only flee, and that even when you flee, the monster sometimes follows.

ATTITUDE?

* * *

Case #4—An aging lady living on her dead husband's military pension was walking home late at night. In order to make the meager military pension meet the rising cost of living, she'd taken a waitress job at an all-night eatery that I often frequented. She'd stopped driving several years earlier due to her aging eyes, and she liked the long walk home in the early-morning chill.

Merrill's Mauraders WW2 (Rangers)

THE COMBATIVE PERSPECTIVE

One fateful night, a teenaged goblin-in-training selected her as his prey. He ran quickly and grabbed her purse. She would not let go, even after he punched her full force in her 70-year-old face. What the hoodlum had not bargained for was that her husband had been a decorated member of Merrill's unit, and he had inculcated in her soul the warrior tradition.

As the cowardly predator cocked his fist back for a second go-around, she slammed a Bic medium-point pen (ironically, it was even red ink) deep into his right eye. This ended the encounter. Little Old lady – 1, Cowardly Goblin – 0. She recovered from her injuries. (The bad guy was later killed in a drive-by shooting.)
ATTITUDE!

* * *

Attitude Is Everything

Here we see four cases, half of them involving nice, domesticated, compliant sheep that were led to slaughter, and the other half involving seemingly defenseless people who turned into fiery dragons and drove away the invaders. I have many similar case studies in my files, some of them extremely sad and others glorious in their humorous apportionment of the justice of the moment.

Interview with a Goblin

In December 1991, I took part in a police action wherein two members of a three-man robbery team were taken into custody after a one-night string of nearly 10 robberies. The third member was shot and killed at the scene in a gunfight with the responding officers.

Some time later I had the opportunity to interview one of the surviving bad guys. He'd been convicted of a number of crimes, including several murders, and was not going to be free for a very, very long time. In short, he believed he had nothing to lose by being honest with me. As it turned out, he was later killed in prison (oh well). The dialogue is taken directly from a tape recording, and hoodlums are not known for their good grammar. (That recording, by the way, is no longer in my possession.) Rather than correct it, I thought it best to leave it as is, so you'd get the full flavor. The following is a word-for-word transcription of my chat with him:

> Author: Do you remember me?
> Robber: Yes, you shot my homeboy.
> Author: You're gonna be gone for a while. I'd like to talk to you about that night. I'm here so I can learn, not to build a case or anything . . . OK?
> Robber: Sure, I'll talk with you. Me and my homeboys wanted to score, so <u>we drove up to the rich neighborhoods.</u>
> Author: There are lots of houses there; how did you pick that one?
> Robber: 'Cause the door was open. It ain't them folks live in South Central; they think they safe and leave their door open for us to come in.

The Combative Perspective

Author: So you found the front door open and just walked in?

Robber: Yes.

Author: Then what happened? Who did you see first?

Robber: We saw the woman. She was nice and smiling like we was they's neighbors. She changed her mind when I put the gun in her face. Her old man was about the same. We tied 'em up right off.

Author: There were a couple of kids, too, right?

Robber: Yes, they tried to hide, but we told 'em we'd bust one on they parents if they didn't come out, and they did. We tied 'em up, too.

Author: Then what happened?

Robber: We wanted the goods—you know, jewels, money, stuff like that.

Author: And they wouldn't tell you?

Robber: Not at first, but after I smacked the woman upside the head with my gun a couple of times, the old man started telling me everything.

Author: How much time do you think you spent in the house?

Robber: 'Bout thirty minutes.

Author: How did you leave—front door, back door?

Robber: The way we came, front door. That was when the old lady across the street saw us and ran inside. I shoulda shot her when I had the chance.

Author: Did you park your car in front of the house

or down the street?

Robber: At least half a block away, but it didn't help this time.

Author: What were you armed with?

Robber: We had Glocks and an Uzi [Author's note: They were armed with four stolen weapons—two Glocks, a Beretta, and a Tec Nine].

Author: Would you have picked that house if you knew that there were armed people inside? You know, armed and ready to shoot it out with you?

Robber: No, we'd have gone to some house with no guns. I been shot before, and I don't want to again.

Author: What do you think you would have done if the woman you first saw had a gun in her hand and pointed it at you?

Robber: I don't know, I might have busted on her (fired at her), or maybe just said, "Hold on, wrong house."

Author: How come you gave up?

Robber: You guys have a rep. You shoot first and ask questions later. I knew that if I didn't lay down, you were gonna bust on me. My homeboy tried to bust on the police, and look at him.

Author: OK, man, thanks for your honesty; good luck.

What were the motivations and attitudes of the criminals, the victims, and the responding officers? What sort of lessons can we learn here?

The Combative Perspective

The lessons inherent in the scenarios above have been repeated with eerie regularity at every event that I have attended, as clear as the Ten Commandments:

1) The dynamics of predator/prey are very similar to those described for police officer encounters: If you look like prey, the predators will try to eat you. If you look like a tough meal, the predators will seek easier prey. This is an important concept that you must give serious thought to.

2) Aggression and even minimal prior planning oftentimes win the day. Predators don't expect their prey to all of a sudden get up and slash their throats in the middle of an assault.

3) Compliance and surrender—although shamefully advocated by some self-serving police groups and some members of academia—often lead to a quick bullet in the back of the head, a lengthy ordeal, or a life-altering axe between the shoulder blades. Surrender is *not* an option.

4) Preparation, however humble, is a key point. If you have no gun, use a knife. If you have no knife, use a steel pipe. If you have no other weapon, use a Bic pen, or spit, but cultivate a spirit of aggression and an affinity for destruction against those who would prey upon you or your family. Be advised: This is so much easier with firearms that it's almost unfair. If

you can't have them, a good blade, or even a nice, sharp pencil, will do fine, albeit with a little more effort. If not, then some good martial arts skills will be better than nothing. Without getting into legalities here, I would caution you to not allow your personal safety to be diminished by artificial directives.

5) When faced with the ultimate test, attitude is everything. An aggressive predator attitude in response to violence is worth more than any weapon.

Appeasement and Compliance

There are those who advocate appeasement and compliance when confronted with a criminal attack. They suggest that you may get hurt if you offer resistance. I can't guarantee that if you resist aggression you will not get hurt, but if you do not, you will probably be injured or worse by the assailants. By not being prepared, you place your fate in the assailants' hands; your future is no longer in your control but in theirs. At least that is what I have seen.

I recall one writer's suggesting that resistance in many cases might be construed as a futile noble gesture. He advised to simply take the beating, the rape, and everything else because at least you'd still be alive afterwards and could be a "good witness." This is the sort of live-coward/dead-hero thing that we have all heard before. The message is to not be a hero because you might get hurt.

The Combative Perspective

It's easy to paint a no-win situation. Real life is rarely so bleak. But we must realize that being a dead hero or a live coward is not the only choice. You can be a live hero or a dead hero, as well as a live coward or a dead coward. My order of preference: live hero, dead hero, dead coward, live coward. Any sort of hero, alive or dead, is better than any sort of coward. And if you are going to be a coward, you may as well have the decency to be dead. And since one day we will all be dead, there are only two real choices: dead hero or dead coward. So the question is, how do you want to be remembered?

This concept of the futile noble gesture is silly. Our freedom was bought and our history written by men who took action against incredible odds. If we must have such a term for action under extreme threat of injury, let's call it HEA, for heroic and exemplary action.

If we had applied the surrender-and-don't-fight attitude to people such as Hannibal, Caesar, Columbus, Cortez, Washington, and a thousand others who have shaped our world with their actions, ask yourself where we would all be. We'd still be living in a cave in Bronze Age Europe.

When faced with violence, the only answer can be greater and overwhelming violence in return. Unarmed? Too bad; that limits your options, but strong hands and a determined heart will still accomplish near miracles.

If it's your time to die—and that is always a possibility, even if you give up without a fight—then meet your destiny with courage and honor and an intent to harm the other side as much as you can. Certainly do not

Victim or Victor? Attitude Is Everything

meet your finest moment like a liberal poltroon with a cell phone hiding under the couch.

This doesn't mean you rush into things like a kamikaze pilot without thinking; rather, you keep your head and deal with the problem coldly and ruthlessly. It can be done. Whether you are armed or not, controlled rage can be a powerful ally—perhaps more so than any mere weapon. Just because it looks bad doesn't mean it's hopeless.

Ask some people what they fear the most, and many will automatically say, "Death." Warriors (and that is exactly what everyone who takes up a weapon in defense is) operate on the very edge of life and death. To be able to truly focus all of your physical, emotional, and mental energy on winning the fight, you cannot allow yourself to dwell on the fear of death. This is a rather involved subject that I hope to delve into in a future volume. Suffice it to say that eliminating the fear of death, as much as is possible, is a worthy spiritual endeavor for any fighter. Most warrior cultures throughout history have also been deeply spiritual and religious ones, far beyond any behavioral codes. We should do likewise.

Home-Defense Realities

Those who've read *The Tactical Advantage* know that I believe it is foolish to go searching an urban structure alone unless you have no other alternative. I can't resist laughing at the antics at some schools that teach single-man clearing as a "school answer" to the

THE COMBATIVE PERSPECTIVE

bump in the night. Single-man clearing is almost suicidal. Nonetheless, there are circumstances where a suicide mission might be the only option, or times when you are just not sure either way. You might elect to go have a "look-see" just to make sure of what that noise was before you commit to call the police at every turn. Also, in the event of an actual home invasion, you'll have the duty to get to all the family members and move them to a safe place. These same principles apply to business defense.

For some, the 12-gauge shotgun is the ideal home-defense/business defense (HD/BD) tool. If you live alone or are the only self-ambulatory adult in the house, it makes perfect sense. If having to get to another family member's room or moving an adult or children to a safe area is not a necessity for you, then keep the shotgun as your primary tool.

If, however, you are a parent, or there are others that you are responsible for "rescuing," you might want to give the pistol a solid appraisal. Consider the tactical need to extract a sleeping 2-year-old out of bed and to a safe room because you have reason to believe there are hostiles breaking in down below! It's not hard to do with a Glock. The same scenario with a souped-up Benelli Super 90 is a different story.

For many people who are forced to live in restrictive environments, a firearm is simply not available. I've spoken to many folks who live in countries where even a worn copy of *Guns & Ammo* will get them brought in for questioning. Yet these laws don't preclude their moral and real need to protect themselves. For them, a big, sharp knife will be a good answer. Remember, something is always better than nothing. If he is able to manage the dynamics of such an encounter, a man with a big knife can often beat a man with a gun. But we'll leave the discussion of contact and edged weapons for another time.

Any home/business defense firearm, short or long, has certain requirements. First, there must be a light mounted to the weapon. Not many invasions that I have investigated or responded to ever took place in broad daylight. In fact, all of them took place after dark. I know all about the Harries and Surefire methods of incorporating light and gun, but if you really want to be effective, get a light mount on your weapon.

The second requirement is a large ammunition supply. This is easier to do with a pistol than with a shotgun, but in either case it's a necessity. This is not intended to somehow "firepower the problem," but instead to make you more tactically versatile. A 29-round magazine in your HD/BD Glock is no big deal. With a shotgun it gets more difficult (where are you gonna hide all those spare shells in your shorts?). Most operators add various ammo-carry methods to their guns, but not without a price. After adding sidesaddles and butt cuffs, the results are guns that are so heavy that Arnold Schwarzenegger would need a chiropractic adjustment after searching an apartment with one!

The Combative Perspective

If we keep drifting back to the slightly modified pistol as the best HD/BD weapon, it's with good reason. Nothing is handier or more maneuverable or allows you more tactical flexibility than a good pistol. The only problem is that you must be good with it.

One method of HD/BD that I've followed at home for years (and when I travel as well) is to put together a "war bag." This is simply a suitably sized belly bag that contains a Glock 24 with a light mount and a couple of high-capacity magazines. There is also an extra light and a cell phone (plus a few other little doom-deliverers that I shouldn't mention in print). This rig can be donned over nightclothes (or lack of same) and will have everything you need to accomplish a hasty HD/BD mission. After the smoke clears and the police are en route, it will also keep the weapon out of immediate sight without your losing control of it.

Tactically speaking, unless there are extreme circumstances dictating a different course of action, you are far better off staying in an ensconced position and allowing the invaders to come to you. If you have protectees to get to, make their room the "safe room" and cease movement once you've arrived to protect them. This is better than moving to retrieve them and then moving again to a different location. Minimize your movements if you can.

Unless you are forced into a hasty rescue, stay in your secure position and announce to the bad guy that you are armed and willing to shoot him and that the police are on the way. If he still comes to get you, he will be in a very poor tactical position relative to that which he would be in if you went to get him. Home and business defense is not difficult to implement, but like anything else tactical, it requires some planning.

When it comes to the uncertainties about how you will react or perform in a life-threatening situation and whether you will become a victim or walk away the victor, remember that in case after case, attitude is the overriding factor affecting outcome.

Part Three
SITUATIONAL AWARENESS

Once we have eliminated uncertainty to the extent that it is possible, awareness of the surrounding environment, or our situational awareness, will be of great importance. Where am I? What is going on around me? Good situational awareness provides ready answers to these questions, allowing you to see the event (or suspect) and analyze the unfolding circumstances before the event is on top of you. This being the case, you can approach it from a position of advantage, rather than being surprised by it.

The Combative Perspective

Lack of situational awareness gets people killed or seriously injured. Some very well-armed and trained individuals have lost their lives due to simple inattention.

Take, for example, the case of William Hickock, the famous Old West shootist. Hickock—one of the best pistol shooters in his day, feared by his colleagues, and winner (not merely survivor, but winner) of numerous gunfights—was shot in the back and killed, by surprise, because he was not paying attention to his environment.

It should be obvious that if we wait to see the other man's muzzle flash or allow him to point his weapon at us, it will probably be too late to do anything about it. When you stop to consider that it takes less than a tenth of a second to press a trigger, an armed adversary takes on a suddenly dangerous character. You see, even if we are very fast, our reactions will never be as fast as his initial action. If we allow him an opening, our life is literally in his hands. The trick is to "react" before he gets his attack fully on the road. In other words, we must act

Situational Awareness

first, and cause him to react to us. If we hesitate, we are truly lost.

Swift reactions are good, but getting ahead of the event is even better. Getting ahead of the event and staying ahead of it is best of all.

The key to good situational awareness lies in *making use* of the presented or available information. This includes not only information about the adversary, but also personal knowledge about your own abilities and your own situation when you see the enemy approaching. With good situational awareness, you begin to project your actions into the future. Instead of the merely adequate insight of "Where am I, and what is going around me," you seek to develop a plan: "Where am I going, and what will I do when I get there?" Simply seeing and being aware of the potential problem at hand is not enough. What you do when the problem begins to unfold is also very important. This is the point in the thought process where most problems develop.

The focus here is be alert, be prepared to act violently, and above all, be willing.

Chapter 5

COOPER'S MENTAL TRIGGER

I first met Col. Jeff Cooper in 1990 when I attended his "basic" pistol course. I had always been a bit more warlike than my fellows in blue, but his lecture on mind-set explained many things. As informative as it was, it was still only a small part of the big picture. While this is not a rehash of his lecture, it does contain a similar message, colored in the lessons I've learned. Cooper's ideas will go a long way toward developing situational awareness.

We cannot anticipate a specific event, so <u>we must anticipate generally</u>. We must develop a state of mind, founded on environmental awareness, where the sudden appearance of a hostile adversary doesn't surprise us. When confronting the enemy, the thought should not be, "Oh my God, is that awful man really breaking

The Combative Perspective

into my house? Is that a real gun in his hand?" Instead it should be, "I see him, he has a gun, and I'm ready for him. Boy, has he made a big mistake!" A predetermined attitude about the confrontation will make all the difference. Technical preparation, aggressive attitude, and situational awareness will save the day!

Most 20th-century human beings, however, are extremely reluctant to harm another person, even when that person has taken clearly overt hostile actions toward them. There are various cultural reasons for this phenomenon, one of which is simply disbelief that another person would really want to hurt us. We cultivate compliance and politeness by placing great societal value on such nice behavior. There is a time for this. But such a mind-set must be overcome when we have to fight for our lives if we want to "live to tell about it."

To do this, you must develop an escalating state of alertness and subsequently an awareness of the environment in which you operate. These will provide you with the ability to respond without hesitation when you are confronted with violence. Additionally, a heightened state of environmental awareness will prevent some of the tragic overreactions that are used by the com-libs (communist liberals—I told you, no punches pulled) in arguing for unilateral public disarmament and generalized neutering.

An excellent method for obtaining such awareness is through intense study of the "Color Code of Readiness." During my earlier research, I learned that the concept of the Color Code of Readiness dates back

Cooper's Mental Trigger

to World War II and the 82nd Airborne. Some years after the war, Colonel Cooper modified it and applied it to the realm of personal combat.

<u>The first mental state is simply unreadiness</u>. This is a state in which you are not attentive at all. All of your focus is within yourself and on your private thoughts and problems, and you are completely oblivious to your surroundings. In Cooper's model, unreadiness is characterized by the color white (it was originally characterized by the color green). Criminals love to come across people in Condition White—they're an easy and tasty meal.

Even if we consider ourselves above it, we may lapse into Condition White when tired or preoccupied. If you are caught in Condition White, your warlike spirit may save you by virtue of your overwhelmingly violent counterattack, but that depends on the bad guy's missing with his first hit.

The next ascending level of alertness is characterized by the color yellow. A man in <u>Condition Yellow is mentally relaxed, but he is aware of his surroundings</u>. He knows what is behind him, as well as anything that appears unusual or out of place. He watches people as he moves throughout his day, whereas a man in Condition White will often have his eyes on the deck. Almost all fights are preceded by subtle clues that a man in Condition White will miss. A man in Condition Yellow will always notice them because he is paying attention. Chances are good that these "clues" might be meaningless, but in the event that

The Combative Perspective

they are a prelude to combat, he is on guard. A man in Condition Yellow realizes that he might have to fight today, but he doesn't know when this will happen or who his enemy will be. The main difference between a man in Condition White and a man in Condition Yellow is that a man in Yellow is paying attention to his immediate surroundings. He may be able to know what he is getting into before it happens by reading the surroundings.

Beyond Condition Yellow, we come to a condition of "specific alert." This is characterized by the color orange. A man in Condition Orange has noticed one of those prefight clues and is specifically alert to its source. He realizes not only that he might have to strike, but that he might now have a specific target. Condition Orange brings us one step closer to the decision to strike. It is relatively easy to shift mental gears from Yellow to Orange, but not from White to Orange. We might not have an "actual human target," but the time of the fight might very well be in the next few seconds . . . even if we haven't actually seen the enemy yet. If we are faced with the reality of our suspicions, we move up the ladder of alertness with a subsequent ease in the decision to shoot. This final level is Condition Red.

Condition Red means that a fight is now quite likely. You haven't decided to strike yet, but you've located a specific individual who might be a hostile and who might require terminal action, depending on his action in the next few seconds.

Cooper's Mental Trigger

Your level of apprehension prior to beginning a tactical problem will also dictate your state of mind during its solution. Be specific with yourself about why you are there and what you are trying to accomplish. Are you simply investigating a suspicious noise, or is it an obvious home invasion? Are you conducting a low-risk administrative perimeter check, or are you hunting for a hidden and armed adversary? Are you dealing with a simple open door that someone forgot to close, or were three armed gang members seen breaking it down seconds earlier? Each of these scenarios is different in their degree of perceived danger. Knowing what you are getting into and what you are trying to accomplish will dictate the tactics you choose.

The determining factor on which your response will be based is a <u>personally established mental trigger</u>. This trigger is simply your perception of the subject's intent based on his actions. It might include a weapon of any sort in his hands, perception of an aggressive move toward you, or, in some extreme cases, an actual shot fired at you.

The mental trigger that you establish is limited only by your legal and moral rules of engagement. <u>You must establish your mental trigger long before the fight</u>, so that when the event unfolds, you will not require a personal debate about whether or not you should hit him. Although the <u>response is a conscious decision, it is</u> almost instantaneous, like a <u>conditioned reflex</u>.

When the fight begins, you must give your undivided attention to solving the problem at hand. This means

The Combative Perspective

simply using proper tactics and shooting well. This requires extreme concentration on the task at hand. You must not dwell on any moves you might have missed with or a faulty tactic that you might have used. Neither do you plan ahead to the next action to be taken. Instead, concentrate on and experience the action you are executing *right now*!

Chapter 6

The OODA Loop

In studying aerial combat in the Korean War, military tactics scholar Col. John Boyd (USAF) noted that the American pilots had a 10:1 kill ratio over the North Koreans. He also noted that the MiG was a faster plane that could outclimb the F-86 of the American forces. He wanted to find out why, if the MiG was in fact a better and faster airplane, the Americans were doing so well against it?

Boyd's studies revealed that one factor contributing to the United States' successes was that we had better-trained pilots. That was not the whole picture, however. The F-86, he learned, allowed dramatically better visibility than the MiG, and it had a set of hydraulic controls that allowed almost instant maneuverability.

The Combative Perspective

Boyd reasoned that the better-trained American pilots could observe their enemy more quickly due to having greater visibility, and they could decide on a course of action more quickly due to good training. Once the course of action was decided, the faster control on the F-86 allowed them to execute maneuvers much faster than the enemy. Thus F-86 pilots had little lag time between observation, orientation, decision, and action. They could operate inside the adversary's response-time envelope.

The natural extension of Colonel Boyd's findings to all areas of personal combat led to the development of a concept known as the OODA Loop, which basically views all conflicts as duels between competitors. In these duels, each competitor Observes his opponent, Orients himself to the opponent and the unfolding events, Decides on a course of action based on that orientation as well as his training and experience, and, finally, Acts out his decision.

Anyone who can move through this loop faster gains a remarkable advantage over his foes by disrupting their ability to respond in a timely or effective manner.

The orientation portion of the cycle is the most important, and the weak point whereby an opponent could penetrate the decision portion.

Each of us bases our decisions on observations of the outside world that are filtered through mental models. Sometimes called paradigms, these mental models orient us to the opportunities or dangers our observations present. In confrontations, an opponent makes

The OODA Loop

decisions based on his orientation to the situation. This orientation changes and evolves because it is formed by the ongoing interaction between observations of unfolding events and mental dialogues that strive to make sense of the situation.

These mental dialogues take two different forms: analysis, or the attempt to understand the observations in terms of existing mental models or patterns of knowledge, and synthesis, or the invention of new patterns of knowledge when existing patterns do not permit the understanding needed to solve the problem at hand.

With faster orientation and action, and through aggressive pressure, it is possible to destroy the adversary's existing mental model (or orientation to the world), as well as deny him the time to synthesize a new one. Aggressive pressure causes indecision, fear, and confusion and overloads the enemy's thought processes, resulting in his inability to cope with the extreme crisis. This promotes compliance and surrender. Thus, it is possible, through sound tactical principles and aggressive pressure on an enemy, to resolve a situation without incident.

Operating within the enemy's decision/reaction portion of the cycle allows you a great advantage in that the mission will be carried out before the adversary can respond, perhaps even before he realizes what is upon him. For example, it can be argued that the Japanese operated within our OODA Loop at Pearl Harbor, just as we operated within Saddam Hussein's OODA Loop in the Gulf War.

The Combative Perspective

With this understanding, we can see that an aggressive operator who initiates the action after proper observation, orientation, and decision will have an overwhelming advantage over a reactive individual. The basic reason is that the aggressive operator's cycle is at the end, or action phase, whereas his opponent's cycle is at the beginning or middle. The aggressive operator has already oriented himself to his opponent (sometimes simply recognizing that he is, in fact, an enemy is enough) and decided on a course of action based on that orientation.

The accuracy of the decision is determined at the orientation part of the cycle by the information available to the operator, as well as how it is filtered and organized. The orientation phase is the most critical part of the cycle, since it shapes the way we interpret the situation.

Everything is based on having good situational awareness that answers the questions of "where am I?," "what is going on around me?," "where am I going?," and "what will I do when I get there?" An unfolding confrontation could be avoided, or it could be overcome unannounced, from such a position of advantage. The concept of the OODA Loop, as applied to police confrontations, has far-reaching implications. It explains why waiting for the other guy to act first is foolishly suicidal, why a man with a firearm in his hand must be handled very carefully, and perhaps some other things as well. This concept could explain how and why a good guy sometimes

THE OODA LOOP

shoots a rapidly turning bad guy in the back instead of in the chest, as intended. It might also explain the nature and source of lag time and how to best overcome it.

If we understand the OODA Loop and apply it, it will work for us and not against us. Moreover, the concept is not in conflict with the core defensive concept (IDOL). If we stay true to the concept of the OODA Loop and use our knowledge of human reaction time to our favor, we've gone a long way toward reducing the dangers of close-quarters confrontations.

VERBALIZING: WHAT DO YOU SAY?

While we're on the subject of using human reaction time to our advantage, I must address a trend that causes me a great deal of concern. I have seen a vast number of students who do a great deal of yelling both before they shoot and while they shoot. I'm not certain, but I suspect someone out there in the training world has been getting very demanding on this "verbalization" stuff. The typical engagement develops with the student "pointing in" on the threat, yelling out some predetermined incantation (presumably powerful enough to ward off civil attorneys), and then (and only then) shooting the hostile aggressor.

With OODA Loops and human reaction time in mind, the idea of reciting some preapproved speech before going into action sounds like an idea invented by some overzealous IA investigator with his brains in

The Combative Perspective

his rear end. Training operators to do this at every engagement is programming them for failure.

Coming from the perspective of the liability-averse culture, I can readily understand the desire to avoid the legal morass, but tactically speaking, verbalizing your intent is fraught with danger. I've never yelled anything at any of the men I've shot, because our roles in life were clearly established at the time of our meeting. An interesting aside is that, in one case, witnesses swore that I'd given the criminal all kinds of commands. Now, before we get into this tachy-psyche stuff, let me tell you that, for whatever reason, I've never experienced time distortion, auditory exclusion, or any of those things, so I really did not yell at him.

In all honesty, there was simply no time to say anything. Had I taken the time to say anything to those men, I would have given them precious seconds (deducted from my own life) to turn the tables on me and kill me.

Tactically, there are two situations that you as an operator might face. One is a confrontation with an individual who has proven, by his actions, demeanor, or armament, that he is a dangerous and hostile aggressor who is not only capable but presently willing to kill you. (Or at least to give your insurance adjuster some serious heartburn!) In this case, you are not required to say anything at all to him. We have all either faced someone like this or heard of individuals like this. They cannot be reasoned with, and attempting to do so will give them the advantage.

The OODA Loop

If you program yourself, through habitual repetition, to always yell before shooting, you are creating several problems. It is difficult, if not impossible, to change a conditioned response in the middle of a fight. Reality tells me that you will probably force yourself to complete your speech before you shoot . . . even if shooting right now is the only thing that will save you.

Although this concept is intended to give an adversary a chance to surrender, in reality, with certain types, it will only present an opportunity to turn the tables on you. A hostile aggressor will hear your yelling (he probably won't understand you) and orient himself to your position, decide to attack, and begin shooting. All of this will probably happen long before you are done with your politically correct and IA-approved statement. Many good guys die every year with cold guns in their hands due to this stuff.

If you do manage to get your whole speech out before you shoot, chances are it will be so rapid and garbled that nobody will understand what you said. All they'll remember is a bunch of yelling and some shots (or was it some shots and a lot of yelling?).

I once worked with a team that had a very liability-conscious team leader. He was more interested in not getting in trouble than in being an effective force ("it's not about enforcement, it's about perception"). He insisted that, upon breaching a door, everyone, from the breacher to the sniper, begin yelling, "GET DOWN! GET DOWN! POLICE! GET DOWN!" I tried to dissuade

The Combative Perspective

him from such a policy, but he insisted that this was the way they had to do it.

A few months later, they ran into some trouble during an entry. It seems that in the dark environment, the residents thought the police entry team was a bunch of rival neighborhood entrepreneurial pharmacists intent on some inventory theft, and one of them actually jumped out of a window. The problem was that it was on the fourth floor! It would have been a funny story, except that the jumper was not actually a bad guy, but rather just a relative of the intended target. The residents and the neighbors (which were actually all very pro-police) remember hearing a bunch of yelling in what sounded like a foreign language. That was an expensive lesson.

OK, what if during the speech/statement you realize that you have to shoot right away? Will you have the presence of mind to stop your chatter to shoot? Most likely you won't, and you'll try to shoot while yelling. Surgical shooting (nothing else is really acceptable in our population-rich cities) requires concentration on the fundamentals of marksmanship. This is difficult enough to do without dividing your attention between your shooting and your speech.

Try this experiment. Set up a humanoid target at seven yards. Now draw your pistol and fire three precise head shots as fast as you can guarantee centered and precise hits. Not hard to do if you understand how to make a pistol work. Now do the same thing again, beginning with a holstered pistol. This time, as the

The OODA Loop

hand touches the pistol, begin yelling the ABCs, and keep yelling until you've fired your shots. I'll bet your second group of shots is much greater in dispersion than the first.

Under stress, you will be about half as good as you really are. So however accurate a shooter you are, you'll be half that good in a real fight just due to the excitement. Add a bunch of needless yelling, and you'll lose another 25 percent.

Remember that I said there were two situations. The second situation is where you are not quite sure whether the man before you is in fact a hostile aggressor. We can paint all manner of "what-ifs," but the point is that you are not sure. This is the time when commands are in order. Nevertheless, a canned statement is certainly not what you want. There are two possibilities here: He could recognize you as a threat and begin firing. He might also simply surrender without your needing to resort to ballistic persuasion.

Anything you say to him should have a specific mission in mind. The goal is to control him and disarm him without unnecessarily exposing yourself to him. The first thing you need is some sort of cover and concealment. Don't just jump out there like Mr. Bullet Sponge and command him to cease. Sneak up into a position of tactical advantage behind something nice and solid. Then make your commands. Don't throw out some IA-approved nonsense ("Please halt in the name of the law, or I will be forced by department policy to take appropriate action in accordance with his highness the chief of police's divinely inspired directives!") Keep your commands short and sharp. Allow yourself enough time to pause and get ready. Similarly, allow the bad guy enough time to comply . . . if he's going to. This way, if the situation allows, you can manage things without taking a life. But you are not overextending yourself tactically for the bad guy's sake.

You must make sure of what you have before you are truly justified in shooting, but when you're sure you are justified, don't give up that advantage by being a blabbermouth. Remember that loose lips sink much more than ships.

WILLINGNESS TO ACT

Part Four

Any student of defensecraft who has followed the discipline of arms for any length of time knows that equipment or skill alone is not enough. The mental attitude you have when you are given the "final exam" has a much greater effect on the outcome than any other factor. Those of you who've read my other works know that I am a vociferous proponent of an aggressive state of mind when the "flag flies."

The only problem is that the flag doesn't fly every day. A shopkeeper in a nasty part of town, or even someone such as a member of a spec-ops

The Combative Perspective

military unit, rarely faces a deadly confrontation in his life. Those who manage to do so time after time are considered rarities. So the problem really becomes one of developing situational awareness. It is a matter of actually anticipating when a fight is either in progress or about to start. A properly conditioned mind and a proper attitude will go far in this department.

The first step in the mental training of a nonvictim is to realize that there are predators out there in the concrete jungle, just as in any jungle. These predators have no regard for your laws, your life, your family, or your possessions. They are out there right now, waiting for you. They will cut off your daughter's finger just to steal her ring, or abuse your wife and beat her to a pulp with as much thought as they'd give to jaywalking. I've met men like this, so don't doubt for an instant that they are out there, right now, in the darkness. They will not show you or your family any mercy, so do not expect any—and when the time comes, do not give any. This is not paranoia. It's reality.

WILLINGNESS TO ACT

The second step is developing the pure willingness to fight with anger, ferocity, and utter ruthlessness when you are offered violence. An old gunfighter once said that it wasn't enough to be accurate or fast, one had to be *willing*. Simply stated, you must be willing, without question or debate, to kill any man who would bring you violence. You must realize that these monsters have no respect or regard for you, so show them the same contempt. You must be willing to offer greater violence in return for violence offered you. That attitude must precede all else. Begin cultivating it now.

Chapter 7

ON COURAGE: REFUTING THE "NEW CONSCIOUSNESS"

Modern domesticated man is an arrogant creature. He assumes that he, in his present form and consciousness, is the norm, and that his ancestors were somehow flawed attempts at creating a perfect and sensitive "Modern Man." This belief that the modern somehow supersedes what came before may be true in terms of technology, but it is not true in terms of humankind or human behavior.

The way man behaves and thinks does not change as easily as we update our computer systems. Man's behavioral characteristics have changed very little, as a matter of fact, since our job description read "hunter-gatherer." It is from these long-gone environments that we get our combative behaviors and attitudes. Our

The Combative Perspective

physiology is developed more for throwing a spear or running down a deer than for firing a rifle or scanning a computer screen.

Before man fought man, he hunted animals for food. There was little emotional response when one of our long-dead ancestors speared an antelope. Well, maybe there was elation and relief that his belly would soon be full, but I'll bet there wasn't much of the Disney-inspired tear-jerking or Bambi-hugging going on. Our combative behavior is something that has evolved from our hunting behavior, and it's grounded in the necessary traits of that hunting behavior.

When you consider the limits of the tools available at that time and the inherent distance limits within which these tools were effective, it becomes quite clear that our ancestors didn't do much sniping. Quite to the contrary, they snuck up on their prey with stealth and cunning and then ambushed it with as much violence as they could muster. This was the same whether they were sticking a deer with a spear or scaring a mammoth off a cliff. In short, we are not programmed to fight at a distance.

As a species, we are programmed and molded for close-interval combat. Although technological advances have allowed us to fight at very long distances, our physiological programming has not quite caught up.

Some experts unknowingly use this disparity in technology and physiology to launch extensive studies in hopes of explaining why only one-third of the men in an infantry squad will willingly and deliberately fire on

On Courage: Refuting the "New Consciousness"

their distant adversaries while the others simply fire into the sky.

One self-proclaimed and well-published expert (who incidentally has never been in combat, much less ever killed another man in that environment) claims that humans are extremely reluctant to kill other humans. Furthermore, he writes that men must be thoroughly desensitized before successfully engaging in mortal combat.

Of course, any high school student of history or archaeology will easily refute that notion, as there is plenty of evidence (hard and documented) that man is not only willing and capable of killing his neighbors, but that he has done so through the ages with efficiency, resolve, and gusto!

The expert cites how animals will never kill another member of their own species as the reason for the human reluctance to kill other humans. The expert tells us that animals will posture a great deal when faced with a member of their own species and that, although confrontations may ensue, there is no specific intent to kill, only to "dominate."

Well, that's true to an extent. When animals are faced with a potential confrontation (nonpredatory in nature), they will do one of four things: submit, flee, posture, or fight. Submission and flight have nothing whatever to do with the combative perspective, so we'll examine the latter two options.

Both the gorilla facing another gorilla and the teenage gang member facing another member of his

The Combative Perspective

gang will bluster loudly and take seemingly aggressive postures. The confrontation with respect to humans will likely be filled with emotional outbursts of profane yelling and so on, and although it might in fact turn deadly, there is rarely actual intent to harm the other. This dynamic exists within members of a group. It is not the same when the opponent is NOT a member of the group. Rather than "posturing," these confrontations tend to be more like actual combat.

When man is confronted by others with whom he feels some degree of relationship, he will usually take the emotionally charged avenue we discussed. This approach allows the operation of any possibly inherent biological or societal inhibitions against killing members of his species. Put a bear and a tiger in the same cage and add a nice T-bone steak as a point of contention, and I don't think there will be much hesitation between the two contenders to harm each other, and perhaps even add the loser to the menu.

During the time when man was open for business as an official hunter-gatherer, he was also running around in tribal units. Anyone not in the tribal unit was probably distrusted initially. Fear of outsiders is not a 20th-century invention. Unlike our modern-day "everything is beautiful, and we are all brothers" society, those were undoubtedly hard days, and there was much competition for survival. If one group had not done well at its hunting-gathering, there must have been great temptation to simply take the bootie from those who had done well.

On Courage: Refuting the "New Consciousness"

Perhaps because of that, man has developed the unique ability to view members of other groups (tribes?) as different. It is almost as if other tribes were seen subconsciously as members of a different species. This allowed an easy bypassing of any emotionally based inhibitions against intraspecies killing and enabled man the predator to evolve into man the warrior.

This pseudopredatory behavior allows man to engage in combat in a manner that parallels the hunting behavior. In hunting behavior there are no emotionally based reactions or inhibitions against killing. Rather, it is a coldly decided and deliberate act once the required parameters are met.

Man has the capability, based on his perspectives in prehistoric times, to engage in combat in either an emotionally aroused state with the resulting stress effects and inhibitions against killing, or in a cool predatory state, which may not have a stress response in evidence and is similar in nature to the hunting behavior.

With regard to the fact that few infantry soldiers deliberately fired on the enemy with the intent to hit them, it could be that there was not sufficient stimulus. The same situation is not evidenced in close-quarters fighting at bayonet point. Perhaps those that did fire with deliberation simply had a greater disposition to the hunter-predator behavior and were thus able to act as predators over a wider range of situations than the rest. This phenomenon can be seen in law enforcement as well. There are officers who have always been reluctant to fire, yet those same officers may be more than willing to "put the stick" to an adversary.

Again, noted experts with no combat experience claim that men who can operate at the nonemotional hunter level are sociopaths. This is simply ridiculous. I suspect that a large portion of men decorated for heroism in combat, members of special military units, and, yes, even a small percentage of police officers fit in that category. To say that all of these men are somehow flawed emotionally and psychologically because they do not fit the experts' fabricated categories is silly.

So how does all this fit in today's world? Motivationally, things haven't really changed in all these thousands of years, have they? Our society has imposed rules on us that prevent preemptive action. That is not as much of a handicap as you might initially think. The resulting defensive-reactive mind-set does make us vulnerable. Remember, aggression is both emotionally motivated and completely uncontrolled or cool, controlled, and pseudopredatory. The choice is clear in terms of effectiveness. The right choice can be trained and developed.

A Final Word

So we know that the savages are out there and we have a burning desire to win should a life-or-death confrontation with one ensue. We have eliminated the uncertainties of battle in our minds, we have developed a keen awareness of our environment, and we are not only ready but willing to utterly destroy any enemy who would stand against us.

What now? Attitude is essential, but so are the tools and the knowledge to use them. Without the tools of war, even the easiest victory may elude the warrior.

Learn the pistol. Learn the knife. Learn the fist. *Develop your ability to fight.* It does not take much more than trying to be a good golfer, bowler, or tennis player. When the final exam comes, however, neither a birdie, a 300 game, nor 40-love will serve you as

The Combative Perspective

well as the combative skills you have at hand. The choice is yours.

Throughout this book, I've tried to get to the meat of what makes one an effective fighter. Overall, I think I've succeeded. These concepts are applicable to everyone in every situation, regardless of their weapons or lack of weapons. Winning a fight, as we've seen, actually has very little to do with what you are armed with and a great deal to do with what you are thinking at the time. This is what is needed to "get your mind right." You've got plenty of material to study and apply.

Here's a quick test to gauge the level of your mindset development and readiness for violence. Right now, this very moment, Hannibal "The Cannibal" Lecter is breaking in through your back door, meat cleaver in hand, hunger in his belly, and murder in his heart! He wants to barbecue you and your kids. What will you do? Where is your Glock?! Where is your Bowie knife?! Even a sharp stick?! Can you get to it in two seconds? One-one thousand, two-one thousand . . .

If you didn't know where your weapon was or you couldn't get to it in time, you are now the dubious recipient of the Distinguished Wooden Cross. The penalty: reread this entire book each night before bedtime, while doing push-ups on broken glass, with your kids sitting on your back . . . for a month. Sweet dreams, young Skywalker!

Good luck!

About the Author

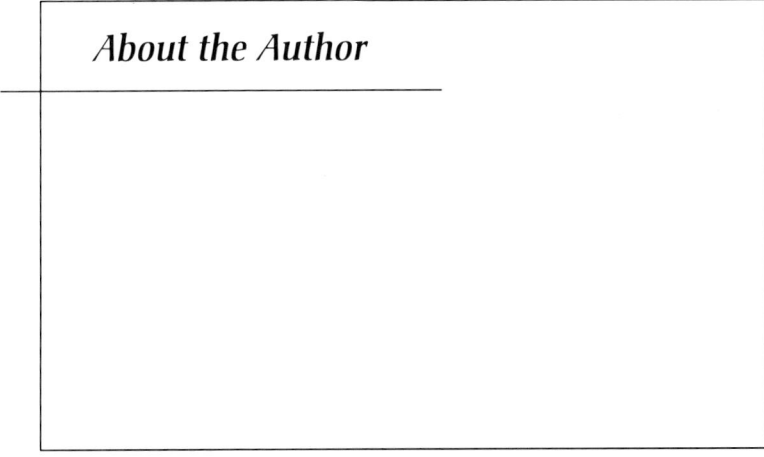

Gabe Suarez is a prolific author in the field of defense and security (www.suarezinternational.com). He served as a police officer in southern California for many years. Specializing in high-risk assignments, he has worked SWAT, gangs, narcotics, surveillance, and single-man night watch patrol.

Suarez is also a lifelong martial artist. He has studied nearly a dozen different systems and has earned several black belt degrees and instructor certifications. He owned and operated his own martial arts organization for many years.

Suarez has written several books and is an internationally recognized trainer and consultant in the field of defense.